Stress-Free
scents
2nd Edition

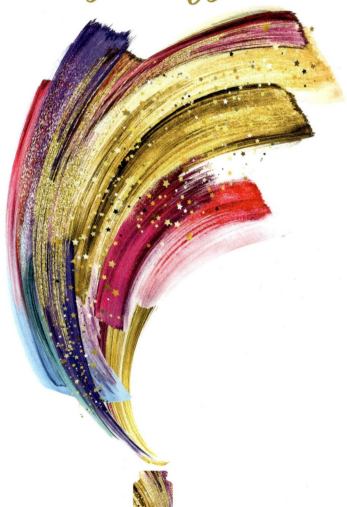

Stress-Free Scents Contents

Welcome...4

Reflex Guide...6

Why Are We So Stressed Out?................................8

What is the Difference Between Stress & Anxiety?.........9

Begin to Win Against Stress and Anxiety.................12

Stress and Essential Oils To the Rescue!................13

Frequent Stress Headaches..................................14

Sleep Interruption...15

Back and/or Neck Pain.......................................16

Feeling Light-Headed and/or Dizzy.......................17

Sweaty Palms or Feet..18

Difficulty Swallowing...19

Frequent Illness...20

Irritability...24

Gastrointestinal...25

Anxiety and Excessive Worry...............................26

Rapid Heart Rate..29

Feeling Overwhelmed...31

Having Difficulty Quieting the Mind.......................32

Poor Concentration...33

Forgetfulness...36

Low Energy...38

Loss of Sexual Desire..40

Welcome To Stress-Free Scents!

Life is just a little better with *Stress-Free Scents*! This guide will help you (and those you love) to start using Young Living's 100% therapeutic-grade essential oils right away to support your everyday wellness.

As you know, essential oils are the "essence" of the plant. They can come from a variety of the plant's parts, and they are mostly extracted through Young Living's unique steam distillation.

The really important thing is that moms and dads all over the world are finding these pure essential oils really helpful in supporting their healthy families. Now you can explore all the ways they may work for you...

Using Essential Oils

Only Seed to Seal®
The recommendations in this book are only good for Young Living's oils that have the Seed to Seal® of approval. These are only the highest-grade oils with the right profile to be effective.

Dilution
Everyone is different, and essential oils are very concentrated. Follow the label on the bottle for dilution. Always start with less essential oil and then add more as needed and as tolerated. Use V-6™ Vegetable Oil Complex for best results. When diluting for babies, use at least 8 drops of carrier oil to 1 drop of essential oil to start. For children ages 2-6 use at least 3 drops carrier oil to 1 drop of essential oil. For ages 7-11 dilute 1 drop of essential oil in at least 1 drop of carrier. After age 12, you can work up to the full-labeled concentration. Consult a health professional before administering oils, especially if your baby or child is sick. Spot test on babies and children before using. Don't use oils with babies in the bathtub, because they may splash and get oils into their eyes and mouths.

Vitality™ Line
So you didn't hear it from us, and we're not supposed to advertise this, but the only difference between a Young Living oil and a Young Living Vitality™ oil is the bottle and the label. The contents are the same. Still, we always recommending reading and following the directions on the bottle...

Topical

Direct Application: Dilute 1 drop of essential oil with 1 drop of carrier oil (50/50) or 1 drop of essential oil with 4 drops of carrier oil (20/80) and apply to affected area. If you feel any discomfort, dilute with more carrier oil such as V-6 Vegetable Complex, fractionated coconut oil, avocado oil, or olive oil.

Neat on Feet: Using the reflex points on the feet (or hands), apply essential oils neat (undiluted) to the energy point(s) that align(s) with your concern.

Internal

Directly Drink: In a tablespoon of milk (including goat or camel), rice milk, almond milk, blue agave syrup, pure maple syrup, or one ounce of NingXia Red® or water add 2-3 drops of oil and swallow the mixture.

Clear Vegetable Capsule: Add 2-3 drops in one side of a 00 veggie capsule. Using a clean dropper, fill the other side with food-grade liquid coconut, olive, walnut, or avocado oil. Marry the two sides together and swallow with 8 ounces of your favorite healthy beverage.

Hand Reflexology Chart

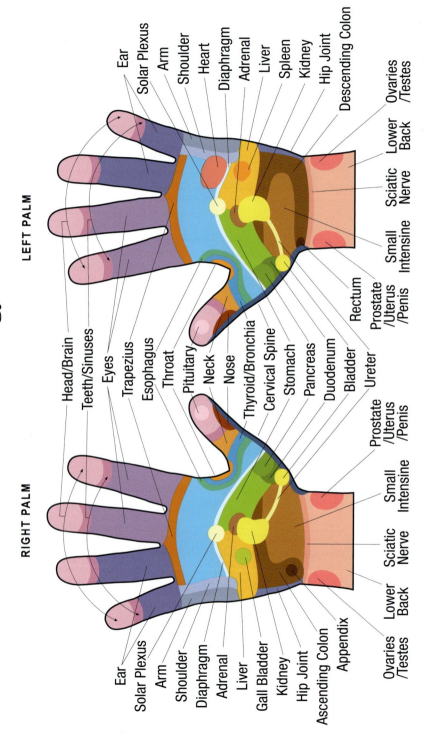

LEFT PALM

Ear
Solar Plexus
Arm
Shoulder
Heart
Diaphragm
Adrenal
Liver
Spleen
Kidney
Hip Joint
Descending Colon
Ovaries/Testes
Lower Back
Sciatic Nerve
Small Intensine
Prostate/Uterus/Penis
Rectum

RIGHT PALM

Head/Brain
Teeth/Sinuses
Eyes
Trapezius
Esophagus
Throat
Pituitary
Neck
Nose
Thyroid/Bronchia
Cervical Spine
Stomach
Pancreas
Duodenum
Bladder
Ureter
Prostate/Uterus/Penis

Ear
Solar Plexus
Arm
Shoulder
Diaphragm
Adrenal
Liver
Gall Bladder
Kidney
Hip Joint
Ascending Colon
Appendix

Ovaries/Testes
Lower Back
Sciatic Nerve
Small Intensine

Foot Reflexology Chart

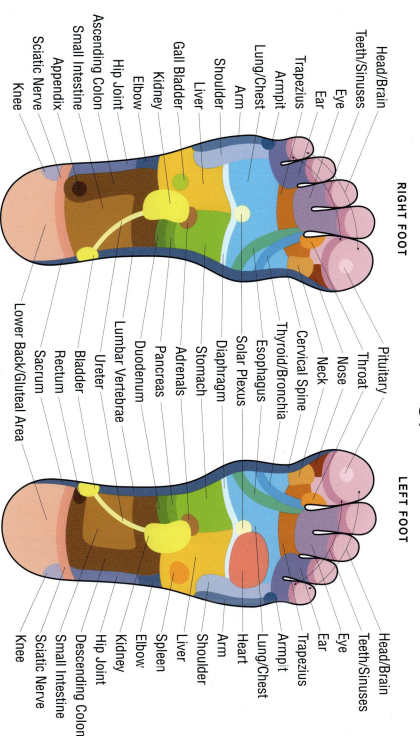

RIGHT FOOT

LEFT FOOT

Head/Brain
Teeth/Sinuses
Eye
Ear
Trapezius
Armpit
Lung/Chest
Arm
Shoulder
Liver
Gall Bladder
Kidney
Elbow
Hip Joint
Ascending Colon
Small Intestine
Appendix
Sciatic Nerve
Knee

Pituitary
Throat
Nose
Neck
Cervical Spine
Thyroid/Bronchia
Esophagus
Solar Plexus
Diaphragm
Stomach
Adrenals
Pancreas
Duodenum
Lumbar Vertebrae
Ureter
Bladder
Rectum
Sacrum
Lower Back/Gluteal Area

Head/Brain
Teeth/Sinuses
Eye
Ear
Trapezius
Armpit
Lung/Chest
Arm
Shoulder
Heart
Liver
Spleen
Elbow
Kidney
Hip Joint
Descending Colon
Small Intestine
Sciatic Nerve
Knee

Why Are We So Stressed Out?

More now than ever people are feeling the stress which leads to anxiety! From adults to children, these disorders are on the rise. Here is what is happening:

- Currently in the United States, anxiety disorders are the most common mental illness, affecting 40 million adults in the U.S. age 18 and older, or 18.1% of the population every year.

- Anxiety disorders are highly treatable, yet only 36.9% of those suffering actually address the issue.

- People with an anxiety disorder are three to five times more likely to go to the doctor and six times more likely to be hospitalized for psychiatric disorders than those who do not suffer from anxiety disorders.

- Anxiety disorders develop from a complex set of risk factors, including genetics, brain chemistry, personality, and life events.

Why is this happening? Well, our 24/7 lifestyle is partly to blame. Phones and social media do not help either.

Stress and anxiety come from many sources such as finances, work, personal relationships, chronic illness, divorce, or moving. Believe it or not, stress is a normal part of life. However, if we don't get a handle on it, there can be real physical and emotional consequences.

Your body automatically jumps into action once a stressful situation is detected. You begin releasing hormones that prepare you to either fight or flight.

What is the Difference Between Stress and Anxiety?

Whether we like it or not, at some point we all will experience stress and anxiety in our lives. Depending on the level of severity, it can have negative impact on your quality of life.

So are stress and anxiety the same? Although stress and anxiety share many of the same emotional and physical symptoms – uneasiness, tension, headaches, high blood pressure and loss of sleep – they have very different beginnings. Determining which one you're experiencing is critical to feeling better and creating a long-term wellness plan.

Generally, stress is a response to an external cause, such as a work deadline or an argument with a family member. However, stress will subside once the issue has been resolved. Because stress is caused by external factors, tackling it head-on is usually the best course of action.

If you're experiencing prolonged, chronic stress, there are many ways to manage and reduce your symptoms, including:

- physical activity,
- breathing exercises,
- essential oils,
- adequate sleep and
- taking time to connect with others.

Anxiety is a person's specific reaction to stress...so it is internal. Anxiety is typically characterized by a "persistent feeling of apprehension or dread" in situations that are not actually threatening. Unlike stress, anxiety can persist even after a concern has passed. In more severe cases, anxiety can escalate into an anxiety disorder, which is the most common mental health issue in the U.S. Anxiety disorders are identified in a variety of ways:

- generalized anxiety,
- panic disorder,
- phobias,
- social anxiety,
- obsessive-compulsive disorder and
- post-traumatic stress disorder (PTSD).

It's important to know how to identify the different signs of stress and anxiety. Stress is a common trigger for anxiety, and it's important to catch anxiety symptoms early to prevent development of an anxiety disorder. We will provide some helpful tips to help support reducing your stress and anxiety!

From the outside looking in, it can be difficult to spot the differences between stress and anxiety. Both can lead to sleepless nights, exhaustion, excessive worry, lack of focus, and irritability. Even physical symptoms – like rapid heart rate, muscle tension, and headaches – can impact both people experiencing stress and those diagnosed with an anxiety disorder. With symptoms that can appear interchangeable, it can be difficult to know when to work on deep breathing and when to seek professional help. In all if these cases, essential oils can help.

In short, stress is your body's reaction to a trigger and is generally a short-term experience. Stress can be positive or negative. When stress kicks in and helps you pull off that deadline you thought was impossible, it's positive. When stress results in insomnia, poor concentration, and impaired ability to do the things you normally do, it's negative. Stress is a response to a threat in any given situation.

Anxiety, on the other hand, is a sustained mental health disorder that can be triggered by stress. Anxiety doesn't fade into the distance once the threat is mediated. Anxiety hangs around for the long haul, and can cause significant impairment in social, occupational, and other important areas of functioning.

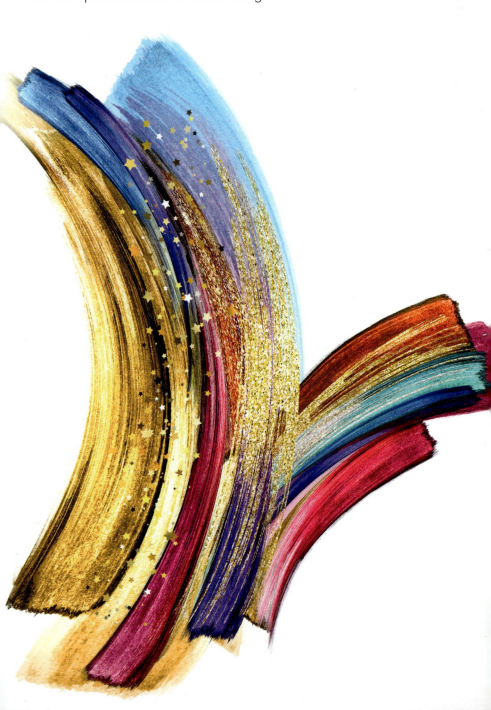

Begin to Win Against Stress and Anxiety

We will get to the essential oils tips for stress and anxiety, but here are some important techniques to utilize to help you win against the stress and anxiety cycle.

It's important to build your own stress reduction toolkit that will include essential oils so that you have more than one strategy to try when stress kicks in.

Let's start with the basics:

• Relaxation breathing - The single best thing you can do when under stress is to engage in deep breathing. Practice this strategy when you're calm so that you know how to use it when you're under pressure. Inhale for a count of four, hold for four, and exhale for four. Repeat.

• Practice mindfulness - Yep, there's an app for that, but the best way to practice mindfulness is to disconnect from your digital 24/7 world and reconnect with your natural world for a specific period of time each day. Take a walk outside and use the opportunity to notice your surroundings using all of your senses.

• Get moving - Daily exercise releases feel-good chemicals in your brain. Making exercise a daily habit can buffer you from negative reactions to stressful events.

• Keep a journal - Writing down your best and worst of the day helps you sort through the obstacles and focus on what went right. It's normal to experience ups and downs on any given day. You can focus on gratitude and that will help to reduce stress.

• Get creative - There's a reason adult coloring books are so popular – they work. Whether you're drawing, coloring, writing poetry, or throwing paint on a wall, engaging in a creative hobby gives your mind a chance to relax.

• Crank up the tunes - Listening to slow, relaxing music decreases your stress response (just as fast-paced music pumps you up for a run).

If you have difficulty managing stress and it impedes your ability to carry out your normal daily activities (like getting to work on time), talk therapy can help. It's important to learn to identify your triggers and responses and find strategies that work for you. Now let's get to the essential oils we love!!

Stress and Essential Oils To the Rescue!

There are a number of emotional and physical disorders linked to stress, including depression, anxiety, heart attacks, strokes, gastrointestinal distress, obesity, and hypertension, to name a few.

High levels of stress can be very unhealthy on the mind and the body. While stress can manifest in many ways, it helps to know a few common symptoms and essential oils that can help to support the reduction those symptoms. Try these different recommendations and use what works best for you and your family.

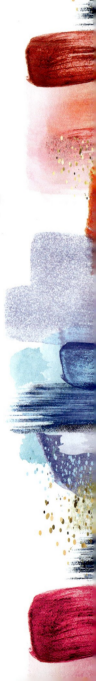

Frequent Stress Headaches

1. Place 1-3 drops of Peppermint essential oil on the back of the neck, temples, under the nose and on top of the forehead. Be careful to keep away from eyes and eyelids.

2. Place 1-3 drops of Peppermint Vitality™ essential oil on the tongue and then push it against the roof of the mouth.

3. Pace 1-3 drops of Panaway essential oil on the back of the neck, temples, under the nose and on top of the forehead. Be careful to keep away from eyes and eyelids.

4. Place 1 drop of Copaiba Vitality™ essential oil on the tongue and then push it against the roof of the mouth.

5. Diffuse this blend of essential oils: 6 drops Peppermint, 2 drops Eucalyptus Globulus and 2 drops Myrrh.

6. Apply 2-4 drops of Stress Away™ essential oil on the bottoms of the feet just before bedtime.

7. Place a warm compress of Tranquil™ essential oil 1-3 drops on the back of the neck or on the back.

8. On the back of the neck, use Deep Relief™ Roll-On.

9. Diffuse these essential oils: 4 drops of Wintergreen, 3 drops of German Chamomile, 2 drops of Lavender, 2 drops of Copaiba, 1 drop of Clove.

Sleep Interruption

10. Add 6-8 drops of Lavender essential oil in a bath to help relax you before you go to sleep. Soak in the tub for 20 minutes.

11. Place 2-4 drops of Lavender essential oil on the bottoms of the feet just before bedtime.

12. Apply 1-3 drops of Peace & Calming® essential oil neat on the shoulders, stomach and bottoms of the feet.

13. Before you go to bed, add 6-8 drops of Roman Chamomile essential oil with ¼ cup Epsom salt in hot bath water and soak until the water cools for 20 minutes.

14. Rub 1-2 drops of Valerian essential oil on the temples and back of the neck several times a day.

15. Place a warm compress with 1-2 drops of Valor® essential oil on the back.

16. Take 1-2 softgels of SleepEssence™ 30-60 minutes before bedtime. Allow for 8 hours of sleep and follow the directions for best results.

17. Take 1-2 tablets of ImmuPro™ before bedtime. Do not exceed 2 tablets in one day.

18. Place 2-4 drops of RutaVala™ essential oil neat to the shoulders, stomach and on the bottoms of feet.

19. Diffuse these essential oils: 12 drops Orange, 8 drops Lavender, 4 drops Dorado Azul, 3 drops Valerian, 2 drops Roman Chamomile.

Back and/or Neck Pain

20. Get a Raindrop Technique® Massage from a Certified Raindrop Technician 2 times weekly or 3 weeks in a row.

21. Apply 2-4 drops of Cool Azul™ essential oil on your back and neck 1-3 times a day or as needed.

22. Use a warm compress with 1-2 drops of Valor® essential oil on the back daily.

23. Apply 2-4 drops of Idaho Grand Fir essential oil on your back and neck 1-3 times a day or as needed.

24. Apply 2-4 drops of Lavender essential oil on Vita Flex™ area of the foot.

25. Take 3 capsules of BLM™ daily with food.

26. Take 2 capsules of AgilEase™ daily with food.

27. Take 2 capsules 2 time a day of Sulfurzyme™ with food.

28. Apply 2-4 drops of Wintergreen neat on your back 1-3 times a day or as needed.

29. Make a blend of these essential oils: 5 drops Wintergreen, 3 drops Lavender, 3 drops Idaho Grand Fir, 2 drops Marjoram. Apply this blend on your back 1-3 times a day or as needed.

Feeling Light-Headed, Faint, or Dizzy

30. Apply 1-2 drops of Peppermint essential oil neat on temples and back of neck.

31. Apply 1 drop of Clarity™ essential oil under the nose.

32. Massage 2-4 drops of Eucalyptus Blue essential oil on the bottoms of the feet.

33. Diffuse Citrus Fresh™ essential oil daily to prevent any lightheadedness.

34. Begin taking 2 packets of NingXia® Red daily.

35. Begin taking Mindwise™ daily and as recommended.

36. Apply 1-2 drops of R.C.™ essential oil on the chest and under the nose.

37. Take 2-3 drops of Frankincense Vitality™ essential oil in a spoonful of water.

38. Take 1 capsule of Peppermint Vitality™ essential oil 2 times a day.

39. Apply a single drop of Dorado Azul essential oil under the nose.

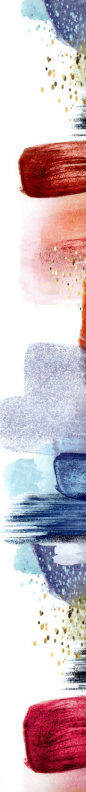

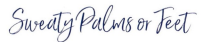

Sweaty Palms or Feet

40. Geranium essential oil was used by the Egyptians to promote beautiful, radiant-looking skin. This oil is also perfect to reduce the symptoms of sweaty palms or feet. Apply 1-3 drops on the hands and feet neat.

41. Apply 1-3 drops of Cypress oil neat to the hands and feet. It also helps with circulation.

42. Apply 1-2 drops of Rose oil to hands and feet.

43. Apply 1-2 drops of Lemon oil with salt to your hands and feet. Rub off after 90 seconds.

Difficulty Swallowing

44. Peppermint oil can be a great oil for esophageal muscle spasms. Take 2 drops Peppermint Vitality™ oil in a spoonful of water.

45. Take 1 capsule of DiGize Vitality™ oil 2 times daily.

46. Take 2-3 drops of Basil Vitality™ essential oil in a spoonful of syrup.

47. Take 2-3 drops of JuvaCleanse® Vitality™ in a spoonful of syrup.

48. Take 2-3 drops of Spearmint Vitality™ in a spoonful of water.

49. Oregano essential oil includes the naturally occurring constituents carvacrol and thymol which can support overall health and maintain a healthy immune system. Diffuse–use it sparingly (just 1–3 drops) and combine it with a complementary oil like Grapefruit, Lemon or Thieves®.

50. Rub 1–2 drops Oregano essential oil on the bottom of the feet or on the back of the neck, but make sure you dilute it with a carrier oil like coconut oil or avocado oil because it can sting on the skin if it's undiluted.

51. Diffuse Thieves® essential oil daily. It is one of my favorite blends to diffuse in the home. Not only does it maintain clean air within the home when diffused, but it also helps to boost the immune system.

52. Apply 1–2 drops of Thieves® essential oil neat on the bottom of feet.

53. Apply 1–2 drops of Thieves® essential oil with a carrier oil like coconut on the back of your neck and wrists.

54. Take a drop or two of Thieves® Vitality™ on a spoonful of honey or coconut oil and swallow. You will want to dilute it when taking internally because it can also feel a bit hot in the mouth. You can also put 1–2 drops in a vegetable capsule and swallow.

55. Ginger essential oil contains a high concentration of gingerol to support the immune system and promote a healthy response to inflammation. Diffuse sparingly (just 1–3 drops) and combine it with an essential oil to complement it like Citrus Fresh™, Raven™, or Peppermint.

56. Apply 1–3 drops of Ginger essential oil diluted with a carrier oil like coconut oil and rub it on the bottom of the feet or the back of the neck.

57. Ginger is a favorite to take internally. Not only is it helpful for the immune system, but it also supports

healthy digestion. Add a drop or two of Ginger Vitality™ Oil on a spoonful of honey or coconut oil and swallow.

58. Put 1-2 drops of Ginger Vitality™ essential oil in a vegetable capsule and swallow.

59. Raven™ essential oil is perfect for fall or winter to help maintain and healthy home and a strong immune system. This is a perfect blend to put in the diffuser. Not only does it make the house smell great, but it helps to maintain clear nasal and breathing passageways and support the immune system.

60. Combine 1-3 drops of Raven™ essential oil with a carrier oil like coconut oil and rub on the chest for healthy breathing. You can also rub it on your neck, feet or muscles after a workout. Adding a few drops to a bath is also very relaxing to the muscles.

61. Lemon essential oil helps to support the body in regular detoxification processes. Lemon oil also helps maintain a healthy lymphatic system which in turn supports the immune system. Lemon is a favorite oil to combine with other oils in the diffuser since it complements almost every other oil or blend and brings a bright cheeriness to the aroma. Diffuse in several areas of the house.

62. Mix Lemon essential oil with a carrier oil like coconut oil and rub on the bottom of your feet, back neck and other areas of your skin. Just be sure not to put lemon oil on your skin and then spend time in the sun right after because it can enhance the effect of the sun on the skin and create a quicker sunburn than usual.

63. Add 1-3 drops of Lemon essential oil in a glass of water to drink or add to a spoonful of honey or coconut oil and swallow.

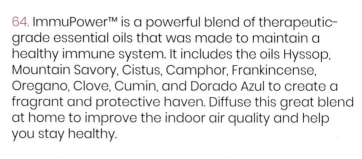

64. ImmuPower™ is a powerful blend of therapeutic-grade essential oils that was made to maintain a healthy immune system. It includes the oils Hyssop, Mountain Savory, Cistus, Camphor, Frankincense, Oregano, Clove, Cumin, and Dorado Azul to create a fragrant and protective haven. Diffuse this great blend at home to improve the indoor air quality and help you stay healthy.

65. Apply ImmuPower™ essential oil diluted on your neck, feet or wrists. It can also be added to the bath or used as a spray.

66. Diffuse Frankincense essential oil to support immune health. You can also combine it with other favorites in the diffuser.

67. Place 1-2 drops of Frankincense essential oil in the palm of your hand, rub your hands together, cup them over your nose and mouth and inhale.

68. Apply 1-3 drops of Frankincense essential oil neat or with a carrier oil to the temples, neck or wrists.

69. Frankincense Vitality™ is an oil you can take internally often to maintain calm and support the immune system. Add you 1-3 drops straight on your tongue or in a spoonful of honey. You can also put 1-2 drops in a vegetable capsule and swallow.

70. Diffuse Tea Tree essential oil to help purify the air and support health. Add other oils as well such as citrus oil, floral oils like Lavender or Geranium, Idaho Grand Fir or Northern Lights Black Spruce.

71. Apply topically Tea Tree essential oil with or without a carrier oil like coconut oil and rub on the feet, nails or on the face to support skin health.

72. Peppermint essential oil a great oil to support the immune system and respiratory system, Diffuse Peppermint essential oil and combine with citrus oil. It helps support healthy breathing and is very uplifting.

73. Combine Peppermint essential oil with a carrier oil like coconut before rubbing on the skin. Apply on the back of the neck, wrists, bottoms of feet and sore muscles.

74. Take 1 drop of Peppermint Vitality™ oil in some water and drink.

75. Diffuse Peace and Calming® essential oil when signs of irritability begin to start.

76. Use Peace and Calming® Roll-on behind the neck and on your temples.

77. Add Peace and Calming® essential oil to your bath and soak for 20 minutes.

78. Orange essential oil can bring feelings of calm, reduce irritability and alleviate anxiety. For the best results, inhalation is the most powerful way to help support irritability. Rub 1-2 drops of Orange essential oil between your palms. Then place your hands in front of your nose and mouth and inhale slowly and deeply.

79. Diffuse a few drops of Orange essential oil in a diffuser throughout the day,

80. Diffuse Ylang Ylang essential oil or apply to the bottom of feet.

81. Place 1-3 drops of Ylang Ylang essential oil on your lower back when you feel irritable.

82. Diffuse Roman Chamomile essential oil to bring emotional balance and stabilize feelings.

83. Apply 1-3 drops of Roman Chamomile essential oil over the throat to reduce irritability.

84. Lavender is soothing and calming. Use Lavender essential oil to help release tension and angry feelings by inhaling straight from the bottle or by rubbing into the back of my neck.

85. Myrrh helps slow down and deepen breathing, helping relax your body and bring mental clarity. Myrrh also reduces headaches and migraines which can increase your anger and tension. Diffuse or use direct inhalation techniques.

86. Bergamot helps relieve stress and irritability by direct inhalation techniques in the palms of your hands.

Gastrointestinal Problems

87. Fennel, Ginger and Cardamom essential oils are great for laxative support. Take any of these oils and gently rub 1-3 drops clockwise over the abdomen.

88. Tarragon and Patchouli essential oils are anti-spasmodic for normal bowel function. Apply any of these essential oils over entire abdomen using soft massage strokes.

89. Lemon and Peppermint Vitality™ essential oils normalize acid balance. Drink 8 oz of water with 1 drop of either Vitality™ oil.

90. Peppermint, Ginger, Lavender, and Basil essential oils are used for general stomach upset. Drink 8 oz of water with 1 drop of any oil, or apply 1-3 drops directly over the abdomen in a gentle massage.

91. Ginger, Peppermint and Fennel essential oils work for occasional gas. Drink 8 oz of water with 1 drop of any oil.

92. Apply 1-3 drops of Ginger, Peppermint and Fennel essential oils directly over the abdomen in a gentle massage. It is safe to apply these essential oils using both methods simultaneously.

93. Clove and Lemongrass essential oils control over-growth of unwanted sugars and other "guests" that may take up residence in your digestive tract: Put 1 drop of each into a vegetarian capsule and take with food.

Anxiety and Excessive Worry

94. Valerian is an herb that has been used since ancient times. It's thought to contain compounds that promote sleep and calm nerves. It can have a mild sedative effect on the body. Add a few drops of valerian oil to a diffuser or inhale directly. Valerian may make you sleepy or relaxed.

95. Add several drops of Lavender essential oil to a bath. Soak for 20 minutes.

96. Inhale Jasmine essential oil directly from the bottle or allow the scent to fill the room through a diffuser.

97. Rub several drops of Jasmine essential oil directly on your ankles and wrists to relieve feelings of anxiousness.

98. Mix 1 drop of Jasmine essential oil, 3 drops of Grapefruit essential oil, 1 drop of Ylang Ylang essential oil, and 4 teaspoons of carrier oil to use as a massage blend.

99. Place a few drops of Bergamot essential oil onto a cotton ball or handkerchief. Inhale the aroma two to three times to help relieve anxiety.

100. Apply 2 or 3 drops of Bergamot essential oil directly to your feet, hands, stomach, or neck where it will be readily absorbed into the bloodstream for symptom relief.

101. Soak your feet in a basin filled with warm water and diluted rose essential oil. You can also add rose oil to your favorite non-scented moisturizer or shea butter and massage into skin.

102. Enjoy a relaxing massage with diluted Vetiver essential oil, or add it to a diffuser.

103. Massage diluted Frankincense essential oil onto your hands or feet. You can also add Frankincense to a diffuser.

104. Inhale Clary Sage essential oil directly when you feel anxious, or massage the diluted oil into your skin.

105. Put 6 drops Clary Sage essential oil and 2 drops of Orange essential oil in your diffuser to reduce anxiety and uplift your spirit whenever you are feeling down.

106. Add several drops of Clary Sage essential oil to your bath water. Inhale deeply to ease feelings of stress and anxiety and lift your mood.

107. Inhale Patchouli essential oil directly or add it diluted to a warm bath or room diffuser.

108. Apply a few drops Geranium essential oil to a cotton ball and waft under your nose a few times.

109. Dilute Marjoram essential oil with a carrier oil and rub into your temples. You may also apply to your wrists or add to a diffuser.

110. Add diluted Fennel essential oil to a warm bath to help relax your body and your mind.

111. Inhale Royal Hawaiian Sandalwood™ essential oil directly from the bottle or by rubbing it into your palms, on your wrists, or on a handkerchief. It is often used before meditation and yoga to foster focus and balance.

112. Apply several drops of Royal Hawaiian Sandalwood™ essential oil directly onto your wrists and ankles to help relieve stress.

113. Use this Anxiety Relief Blend by mixing 6 drops of Sandalwood essential oil, 2 drops of Rose essential oil, and 4 teaspoons of carrier oil. Use the blend as a full body massage oil.

114. Rub several drops of Ylang Ylang essential oil directly on your feet, neck, wrists, and back to reduce feelings of anxiety.

115. Diffuse this Anxiety Relief Blend by mixing 1 drop Clary Sage oil, 1 drop of Ylang Ylang oil, 2 drops of Lavender essential oil, and 4 teaspoons of carrier oil, and use it as a massage blend.

116. Add several drops of Frankincense essential oil to your bath water. Inhale deeply and allow the stress to melt away.

117. Use this Anxiety Relief Blend by mixing 4 drops of Frankincense essential oil, 2 drops of Lemon essential oil, 4 drops of Jasmine essential oil, and 4 teaspoons of carrier oil to make the perfect massage oil blend.

118. Chamomile essential oil can be inhaled straight from the bottle to soothe the nervous system.

119. Chamomile may be diffused using a room diffuser to promote calm and peace.

120. Diluted chamomile essential oil can be massaged directly into the skin or added to a warm bath to experience relief from anxiety.

121. Orange essential oil is one of the best essential oils to use in a diffuser if you wish to remove anxiety and uplift your mood. It's also valuable for improving concentration and boosting energy levels.

122. Orange essential oil can be inhaled directly from the bottle or from the palms of your hands to relieve anxiety and to get an instant mood lift.

123. Use this Anxiety Relief Blend by mixing 6 drops of Orange essential oil, 2 drops of Lavender essential oil, and 3 teaspoons of carrier oil. Use as a full body massage oil.

124. Blend 10 -20 drops each of: Cypress, Helichrysum, Lavender, Marjoram, Frankincense. Apply topically to heart, reflex points on feet and wrists.

125. Blend 10 -20 drops each of: Lavender, Orange, Ylang Ylang. Apply topically to heart, reflex points on feet and wrists.

126. Diffuse 4 drops of Copaiba, 3 drops of Orange and 2 drops of Frankincense.

– Muscle Tension –
You can use each of these oils separately or layer them to create your own blend. Use 1-3 drops with a carrier oil when you apply topically to the area of tension.

127. Peppermint essential oil contains menthol, which has a cooling effect on sore, achy muscles. It also has analgesic, antispasmodic, and anti-inflammatory properties.

128. Helichrysum essential oil relieves muscle spasms, inflammation, and pain.

129. Marjoram essential oil relaxes muscle spasms and tension. It's known for its ability to ease pain and inflammation.

130. Lavender essential oil is prized for its ability to calm and relax. It also relieves pain and inflammation.

131. Eucalyptus essential oil. Eucalyptus has a cooling effect on muscles and reduces pain and inflammation.

132. Roman and German Chamomile essential oils can help with pain and inflammation. They also help soothe muscle tension and reduce spasms.

133. Rosemary essential oil is noted for its ability to ease pain and inflammation.

134. Cypress essential oil calms and relaxes muscles spasms and works to soothe inflammation.

135. Sandalwood essential oil alleviates muscle spasms, tension, and inflammation.

136. Ginger essential oil has a warming effect on sore muscles, which helps relieve pain.

137. Black Pepper essential oil alleviates pain by warming up your body.

138. Clove essential oil is often used to treat pain. It also has a warming effect on sore muscles.

139. Clary Sage essential oil alleviates muscle tension and spasms while promoting relaxation.

140. Juniper essential oil eases tension and eliminates muscle spasms.

141. Lemongrass essential oil works quickly to reduce inflammation and swelling.

142. Wintergreen essential oil is derived from a plant that contain high amounts of methyl salicylate, which contains pain-relieving qualities similar to aspirin. Its therapeutic properties make it effective for relieving muscle and joint pain.

143. Vetiver essential oil has anti-inflammatory properties including the ability to reduce swelling, especially in the joints.

144. Copaiba essential oil has both analgesic and anti-inflammatory properties, some of which have been shown to reduce the body's natural response to pain.

Feeling Overwhelmed

145. Diffuse 3 drops of Frankincense, 3 drops of Bergamot and 3 drops of Lavender essential oils.

146. Diffuse 4 drops of Lavender, 3 drops of Roman Chamomile and 2 drops of Ylang Ylang essential oils.

147. Diffuse 5 drops of Frankincense, 2 drops of Melissa and 2 drops of Patchouli essential oils.

148. Diffuse 3 drops of Cedarwood, 3 drops of Bergamot and 2 drops of Lime essential oils.

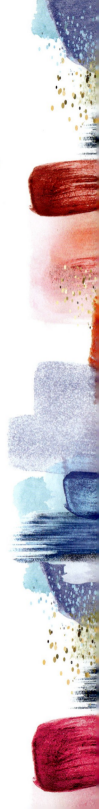

Having Difficulty Quieting the Mind

149. To quiet the mind, rub Lavender essential oil behind the ears before going to bed.

150. Diffuse Lavender essential oil by your bed to experience the healing effects of lavender at night.

151. Combine five drops of Rose essential oil and five drops of Lavender in a diffuser. You can put the diffuser in your bedroom to inhale at night to quiet the mind or in the living room to experience the healing benefits while watching TV and unwinding after a long day at work.

152. If a restless mind is keeping you awake at night, Jasmine essential oil's sedative effects can be just what you need. Unlike other essential oils, Jasmine doesn't need to be diluted. It works well in full concentration. It can be applied topically during a massage or diffused.

153. Roman Chamomile essential oil has sedative properties that help relax the mind. It's one of the most popular essential oils for anxiety, and studies confirm its mental health benefits. Diffuse five drops or inhale directly from the bottle.

154. Rub 1-2 drops of Roman Chamomile essential oil on your temples.

155. Geranium essential oil is packed with powerful healing properties. Along with being a natural antiseptic, it helps people who suffer from their mind never shutting off. Place 1 drop in the palm of your hands, rub your hands together and cup them over nose. Breathe in slowly.

156. Rub 2-3 drops of Bergamot essential oil into your hands and cup your mouth and nose. Slowly breathe in the oil.

157. Add a few drops of Frankincense essential oil to calm the mind and relax.

Poor Concentration

158. Vetiver is grounding, calming, and stabilizing. Apply 1-2 drops on the bottom of feet or inhale for a few minutes in the morning and at bedtime.

159. Vetiver used in combination with Lavender and Cedarwood (1-2 drops on the bottom of feet, especially the big toe – a Vita Flex point to the brain).

160. Lavender is a great aid for relaxing and winding down before bedtime, and provides balancing properties. Apply 1-2 drops to the neck and feet before bedtime, add to a diffuser or use in combination with Vetiver and Cedarwood on the bottom of feet.

161. Rosemary smells so good. It's soothing scent both helps to reduce mental fatigue and helps to uplift... so it's great when you have the afternoon slump and need to wake up. Rosemary is great for helping with mental focus. Apply 1-2 drops with a carrier oil on the back of the neck and hairline, or add to the diffuser.

162. Peppermint is one of the best oils to use for focus and concentration. The minty aroma stimulates the mind and gives a boost of energy. Add 6 drops each of Peppermint and Lemon together for the best diffuser blend when you need to get things done.

163. Like Rosemary, Basil has an herbaceous scent that's so soothing. Pair with a citrus oil like Lemongrass to help uplift and get you going, while Basil helps you to chill. Add 6 drops each of Basil and Lemongrass to a diffuser while you're working on a project.

164. Lemongrass has a refreshing, clean scent that helps to motivate when you're on deadline for a project. Use in combination with Basil or Rosemary for an uplifting aroma. Use 6 drops each of Lemongrass and Basil/Rosemary in the diffuser.

165. Frankincense is one of the best essential oils for grounding and focus. Put a 1-2 drops behind the neck and on the temples. It's gentle so you don't have to

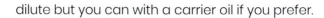

dilute but you can with a carrier oil if you prefer.

166. Lemon has an uplifting scent that's great alone to get motivated to get things done, or pair with Peppermint for an invigorating aroma in the diffuser. Add 6 drops each in the diffuser.

167. Cypress is an herbaceous oil that's great for grounding and calming. It's great when you're feeling overwhelmed about a project or deadline. Pair it with a citrus oil like Bergamot or Lemon in the diffuser. Use 6 drops of each in the diffuser.

168. Bergamot is a citrus oil that's uplifting and invigorating like Lemon. Use it alone in the diffuser or pair with Patchouli in the diffuser. Add 6 drops of each to the diffuser.

169. Patchouli is a popular oil for calming and relaxing, which is perfect when you've been putting off an assignment or project. Pair it with a citrus oil like Bergamot to get motivated to get tasks done.

170. Clarity™ is an oil blend (Basil, Peppermint, Rosemary, Geranium, Coriander, Ylang Ylang, Bergamot, Lemon, Jasmine and Roman Chamomile) with both citrus and herbaceous oils that help with mental alertness and gives clarity. It's the perfect oil blend to stay on task and get things done. Put 10 drops in the diffuser, or mix 1-2 drops with carrier oil and apply to the temples.

171. Peace and Calming® is an oil blend (Tangerine, Orange, Ylang Ylang, Patchouli and Blue Tansy) helps uplift the spirit, promoting relaxation and a deep sense of peace. Apply 1-2 drops with a carrier oil on the feet morning and at bedtime, inhale for a few minutes in the morning and night or add to a diffuser at bedtime.

172. Brain Power™ is an oil blend (Sandalwood, Cedarwood, Melissa, Frankincense, Blue Cypress, Lavender and Helichrysum) can be used to clarify thoughts and develop greater focus. Apply 1-2 drops with a carrier oil on the back of the neck in the

morning and at bedtime, inhale for a few minutes in the morning and night or add to a diffuser at bedtime.

173. Blend 5 drops Vetiver, 5 drops Valor, 5 drops Cedarwood, 5 drop Lemon and 5 drops Lavender essential oil and diffuse away!

174. Blend 1 drop Sandalwood, 1 drop Cinnamon Bark and 2 drops Frankincense in a diffuser or inhale the blend directly.

175. Blend 7 drops Frankincense, 3 drops Rosemary, 2 drops Eucalyptus, and 3 drops Cardamom in a diffuser or inhale the blend directly.

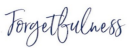

Forgetfulness

176. Diffuse Cedarwood essential oil or apply 1-2 drops on temples or back of neck or on the Vita Flex brain points on the feet 1-2 times a day.

177. Diffuse Clarity essential oil or apply 1-2 drops on the temples or back of neck or on the Vita Flex brain points on the feet 1-2 times a day.

178. Diffuse Sacred Frankincense essential oil or apply 1-2 drops on the temples or back of neck or on the Vita Flex brain points on the feet 1-2 times a day.

179. Diffuse Roman Chamomile essential oil or apply 1-2 drops on the temples or back of neck or on the Vita Flex brain points on the feet 1-2 times a day.

180. Diffuse Rosemary essential oil or apply 1-2 drops on the temples or back of neck or on the Vita Flex brain points on the feet 1-2 times a day.

181. Diffuse Idaho Grand Fir essential oil or apply 1-2 drops on the temples or back of neck or on the Vita Flex brain points on the feet 1-2 times a day.

182. Diffuse Peppermint essential oil or apply 1-2 drops on the temples or back of neck or on the Vita Flex brain points on the feet 1-2 times a day.

183. Apply Brain Power™ essential oil on the Vita Flex brain points on the feet 1-2 times daily.

184. Apply Common Sense™ essential oil on the Vita Flex brain points on the feet 1-2 times daily.

185. Apply 1-2 drops of Valor® on the temples or back of neck or on the Vita Flex brain points on the feet 1-2 times a day.

186. Take MindWise™ daily as directed.

187. Take PD 80/20™ daily as directed.

188. Take NingXia Red® daily as directed.

189. Take Sulfurzyme™ daily as directed.

190. Take Essentialzyme™ daily as directed.

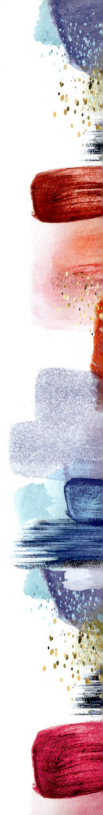

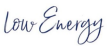

Low Energy

191. Apply 2-4 drops of diluted Peppermint essential oil on temples and behind the ears 2-4 times a day as needed.

192. Apply 2-4 drops of diluted Awaken™ essential oil on temples and behind the ears 2-4 times a day as needed.

193. Apply 2-4 drops of diluted Motivation™ essential oil on temples and behind the ears 2-4 times a day as needed.

194. Apply 2-4 drops of diluted Lemongrass essential oil on temples and behind the ears 2-4 times a day as needed.

195. Apply 2-4 drops of diluted Eucalyptus Blue essential oil on temples and behind the ears 2-4 times a day as needed.

196. Apply 2-4 drops of Valor® essential oil on temples and behind the ears 2-4 times a day as needed.

197. Use Orange essential oil to lower cortisol levels, uplift your mood, and instantly boost your energy.

198. Lemon essential oil is another citrus essential oil that helps with energy and is a favorite. Lemon's zesty and upbeat aroma is inspiring and makes you feel good and energized. Simply add 1-2 drops of Lemon on a tissue and inhale.

199. Rosemary essential oil contains Cineole, a potent energy boosting agent. According to one study, Cineole provides positive stimulatory effects that help to boost moods and fight low energy. Diffuse or inhale 1-2 drops directly.

200. Basil essential oil acts as a stimulant reducing sluggishness and making you more alert. Just inhale your Basil oil for that energy boost when you need it.

201. Inhaling Juniper essential oil can help reduce the physical, emotional and mental fatigue that's weighing you down. The scent stimulates warmth and improves your energy levels.

Loss of Sexual Desire

202. Apply 4-6 drops of diluted 50;50 Jasmine essential oil on neck, shoulders and lower abdomen 1-3 times a daily.

203. Apply 4-6 drops of diluted 50;50 Ylang Ylang essential oil on neck, shoulders and lower abdomen 1-3 times a daily.

204. Apply 4-6 drops of diluted 50;50 Nutmeg essential oil on neck, shoulders and lower abdomen 1-3 times a daily.

205. Apply 4-6 drops of diluted 50;50 Rose essential oil on neck, shoulders and lower abdomen 1-3 times a daily.

206. Apply 4-6 drops of diluted 50;50 Clary Sage essential oil on neck, shoulders and lower abdomen 1-3 times a daily.

207. Apply 4-6 drops of diluted 50;50 En-R-Gee™ essential oil on neck, shoulders and lower abdomen 1-3 times a daily.

208. Apply 4-6 drops of diluted 50;50 Joy® essential oil on neck, shoulders and lower abdomen 1-3 times a daily.

209. Apply 4-6 drops of diluted 50;50 Valor® essential oil on neck, shoulders and lower abdomen 1-3 times a daily.

210. Use Progessence Plus™ as recommended on the label.

211. Use EndoGize™ as recommended on the label.

212. Use Mineral Essence™ as recommended on the label.

213. Use PD 80/20™ as recommended on the label.

214. Use ImmuPro™ as recommended on the label.

215. Use Super B™ as recommended on the label.

Symptoms of stress can vary and change over time. Knowing your own responses to stress can help you increase awareness of how stress manifests for you. Recognizing this vital information will help you learn to use stress reduction techniques at the first signs of stress to avoid long-term repercussions.

You also have essential oils to help you along the way. Try the different recommendations in this book to see what works best for you and how to improve your own wellness. Essential oils are powerful and natural. They can provide the support you are looking for on a long-term basis.